THE ULTIMATE GALVESTON DIET

Comprehensive Solution for Healthy Weight Loss and Stabilize Hormonal Balance.

Michael Junior

Copyright©2023 Michael Junior

TABLE OF CONTENT

INTRODUCTION

"The Ultimate Galveston Diet," a complete revolutionary solution meant to rethink your approach to weight loss and hormone balance. In a world flooded with diet programs, ours distinguishes out as a comprehensive, science-backed strategy that goes beyond calorie monitoring.

This diet is tailored to your specific goals, whether you're looking to lose weight, achieve hormonal balance, or improve your general well-being.

The Galveston Diet is more than simply a collection of rules; it's a way of life that includes fueling your body, balancing hormones, and cultivating long-term habits.

This program was created with the goal of empowering women in mind, and it is inspired by the dynamic coastal energy of Galveston, Texas, which embodies a sense of rebirth, vitality, and balance.

Our method is based on the realization that hormonal variations can have a substantial influence on weight control. This diet strives to establish a harmonious environment within the body, supporting healthy weight reduction and promoting long-term well-being, with a strong emphasis on enhancing hormonal health.

The Ultimate Galveston Diet puts you on a path toward a healthier and more vibrant self by combining healthy and tasty food planning, focused workouts, and mindful practices.

Say goodbye to restricted diets and welcome to a sustainable lifestyle that nourishes your body as well as your hormonal balance.

Join us on this revolutionary journey, where every meal, activity, and self-care practice is a step toward reaching your health and wellness objectives.

The Ultimate Galveston Diet is more than a regimen; it's an invitation to adopt a complete and balanced lifestyle that will help you to reach your greatest potential and live a vibrant existence. Let the adventure begin!

Quinoa Salad with Roasted Vegetables and Avocado

Ingredients:
- 1 cup quinoa, rinsed
- 2 cups mixed vegetables (zucchini, cherry tomatoes, bell peppers)
- 1 tablespoon olive oil
- Salt and pepper to taste
- 1 avocado, sliced
- 1/4 cup feta cheese, crumbled (optional)
- Fresh herbs (such as parsley or cilantro), chopped

Preparation:
1. **Preheat the Oven:**
   - Preheat the oven to 400°F (200°C).

2. **Roast Vegetables:**
   - Toss the mixed vegetables with olive oil, salt, and pepper.

   - Spread them on a baking sheet and roast in the preheated oven for 20-25 minutes or until golden brown and tender.

3. **Cook Quinoa:**
   - While the vegetables are roasting, cook the quinoa according to package instructions. Typically, bring 2 cups of water to a boil, add the quinoa, cover, and simmer for 15-20 minutes until cooked.
   -

4. **Assemble the Salad:**
   - In a large bowl, combine the cooked quinoa and roasted vegetables.
   - Gently fold in the sliced avocado, crumbled feta cheese (if using), and fresh herbs.

5. **Season to Taste:**
   - Adjust the seasoning with salt and pepper according to your taste preferences.

6. **Serve:**
   - Serve the quinoa salad in bowls, garnished with extra fresh herbs and a drizzle of olive oil if desired.

Benefits:
1. **Nutrient-Dense:** This salad is rich in vitamins, minerals, and antioxidants from the colorful vegetables and fresh herbs.

2. **Protein-Packed:** Quinoa is a complete protein, providing all essential amino acids, making this salad suitable for vegetarians and vegans.

3. **Healthy Fats:** Avocado contributes heart-healthy monounsaturated fats, promoting satiety and overall well-being.

4. **Fiber-Rich:** Both quinoa and vegetables are excellent sources of fiber, supporting digestive health and weight management.

5. **Low-Processed:** By using whole, unprocessed ingredients, this recipe minimizes the intake of refined and processed foods, promoting a clean and wholesome diet.

Application:
- Ideal for a quick and nutritious weeknight dinner.
- Perfect for meal prepping lunches, as the salad can be refrigerated and enjoyed the next day.

- Great for potlucks, picnics, or as a side dish at gatherings, providing a healthier alternative to traditional options.

This recipe showcases the beauty of whole, unprocessed foods, offering a delicious and satisfying meal that nourishes your body with essential nutrients.

Relaxing Chamomile Lavender Tea

Ingredients:

- 1 chamomile tea bag
- 1/2 teaspoon dried lavender buds (culinary grade)
- 1 teaspoon honey (optional)
- 1 slice of lemon (optional)

Preparation:

1. **Boil Water:**
   - Bring a cup of water to a boil.

2. **Prepare Tea Infusion:**
   - Place the chamomile tea bag and dried lavender buds in a teapot or a heatproof mug.

3. **Pour Hot Water:**
   - Pour the boiling water over the tea bag and lavender buds.

4. **Steep:**
   - Let the tea steep for 5-7 minutes to allow the flavors to infuse.

5. **Strain:**
   - If using loose lavender buds, strain the tea to remove them.

6. **Sweeten and Garnish:**
   - Add honey to taste, and garnish with a slice of lemon if desired.

7. **Enjoy Mindfully:**
   - Find a quiet space, sip the tea slowly, and focus on the calming aroma and flavors.

Benefits:
1. **Calming Herbs:** Chamomile is known for its calming properties, while lavender is recognized for its stress-relieving and sleep-promoting effects.

2. **Mood Enhancement:** The act of sipping a warm, aromatic tea can have a positive impact on mood, reducing feelings of stress and anxiety.

3. **Hydration:** Staying hydrated is crucial for overall well-being, and opting for herbal teas is a healthier alternative to sugary or caffeinated beverages.

4. **Natural Relaxant:** Lavender has natural compounds that can act as mild sedatives, promoting relaxation and reducing tension.

5. **Mindful Ritual:** The process of preparing and enjoying the tea can become a mindful ritual, fostering a sense of calm and tranquility.

Application:

- Incorporate this tea into your evening routine to signal the transition from a busy day to a restful evening.

- Enjoy it before bedtime to enhance relaxation and improve sleep quality.

- Share this calming ritual with friends or family during social gatherings for a serene and pleasant experience.

This Relaxing Chamomile Lavender Tea serves as a simple yet effective tool for stress management, offering a comforting and natural way to unwind and find peace in the midst of a hectic day.

Energizing Morning Workout Routine

Ingredients:
- Comfortable workout attire
- Athletic shoes
- Exercise mat
- Water bottle

Preparation:
1. **Warm-Up (5 minutes):**
   - Start with light cardio, such as jumping jacks or a brisk walk in place, to increase your heart rate and warm up your muscles.

2. **Strength Training (15 minutes):**
   - Perform bodyweight exercises like squats, lunges, push-ups, and planks to engage major muscle groups.

3. **Cardiovascular Exercise (15 minutes):**
   - Incorporate cardio activities like jogging in place, high knees, or jumping rope to elevate your heart rate and improve endurance.

4. **Flexibility and Stretching (10 minutes):**
   - Dedicate time to stretching exercises, focusing on each muscle group to improve flexibility and reduce the risk of injury.

5. **Cool Down and Relaxation (5 minutes):**
   - Finish with gentle movements and deep breathing exercises to cool down and promote relaxation.

Benefits:
1. **Mood Enhancement:** Regular exercise releases endorphins, promoting a positive mood and reducing stress and anxiety.

2. **Improved Cardiovascular Health:** Cardio exercises strengthen the heart and improve circulation, benefiting overall cardiovascular health.

3. **Weight Management:** Combining strength training and cardio helps burn calories, aiding in weight management and body composition.

4. **Enhanced Flexibility:** Stretching exercises increase flexibility, preventing

muscle stiffness and improving range of motion.

5. **Increased Energy Levels:** Engaging in regular physical activity boosts energy levels, making you feel more alert and ready to tackle the day.

Application:

- **Morning Routine:** Incorporate this workout into your morning routine for an energizing start to the day.

- **Lunch Break Workout:** If mornings are hectic, use your lunch break for a quick exercise session to re-energize for the afternoon.

- **Family Fitness:** Involve family members or friends for a group workout, making it a fun and social activity.

- **Consistency is Key:** Aim for at least 3-5 sessions per week to experience the full benefits of regular exercise.

This Energizing Morning Workout Routine serves as a recipe for a healthier and more active lifestyle.

It's a versatile and accessible way to integrate regular exercise into your daily routine, promoting physical and mental well-being.

Balanced Day Meal Timing Plan

Ingredients:
- Water
- Nutrient-dense foods (vegetables, fruits, lean proteins, whole grains)
- Healthy fats (avocado, nuts, olive oil)

Preparation:
1. **Morning Boost (7:00 AM):**
   - Start your day with a glass of water to rehydrate your body.

   - Have a balanced breakfast with a mix of protein, fiber, and healthy fats. For example, oatmeal with berries and a sprinkle of nuts.

2. **Mid-Morning Snack (10:00 AM):**
   - Stay hydrated with water or herbal tea.

   - Snack on a piece of fruit or a small handful of nuts to maintain energy levels.

3. **Lunch (1:00 PM):**
   - Consume a well-rounded lunch containing lean protein, whole

grains, and plenty of vegetables. A grilled chicken salad with quinoa and a variety of veggies is a nutritious option.

4. **Afternoon Pick-Me-Up (3:00 PM):**
   - Hydrate with water or green tea.

   - Choose a light and protein-rich snack, like Greek yogurt with honey or a handful of edamame.

5. **Pre-Workout Fuel (5:30 PM):**
   - Drink water to stay hydrated.

   - Have a small snack that combines carbohydrates and protein, such as a banana with almond butter, before your workout.

6. **Dinner (7:30 PM):**
   - Opt for a balanced dinner with lean protein, vegetables, and a serving of healthy carbs. Baked salmon with roasted sweet potatoes and steamed broccoli is a nutritious choice.

7. **Evening Snack (9:00 PM):**
   - Hydrate with water or a calming herbal tea.

- If hungry, choose a small and light snack, such as a handful of cherry tomatoes or a slice of whole-grain toast with avocado.

Benefits:
1. **Stable Energy Levels:** By spacing meals and snacks throughout the day, you maintain a steady supply of nutrients, preventing energy crashes.

2. **Improved Metabolism:** Regular meal timing helps regulate your metabolism, promoting efficient calorie burning.

3. **Nutrient Absorption:** Breaking your daily intake into multiple meals allows for better nutrient absorption and utilization.

4. **Balanced Nutrition:** Ensuring a mix of proteins, carbohydrates, fats, and micronutrients supports overall health and well-being.

5. **Sustained Focus and Productivity:** Consistent nutrition supports mental clarity and focus, contributing to productivity throughout the day.

Application:

- Customize the meal timings based on your daily schedule and preferences.

- Adjust portion sizes based on individual nutritional needs and activity levels.

- Make this Balanced Day Meal Timing Plan a guideline rather than a strict rule, allowing for flexibility and enjoyment in your eating habits.

This Balanced Day Meal Timing Plan serves as a recipe for a well-fueled and energized day. It's a flexible guide to help you establish a routine that supports your nutritional needs and overall health.

Mindful Eating Meditation Bowl

Ingredients:
- 1 cup cooked quinoa
- 1/2 cup steamed broccoli florets
- 1/2 cup sliced carrots
- 1/4 cup diced avocado
- 1/4 cup cherry tomatoes, halved
- 2 tablespoons sesame seeds
- Fresh cilantro for garnish

Preparation:
1. **Prepare Ingredients:**
   - Cook the quinoa according to package instructions.

   - Steam the broccoli and carrots until tender but still vibrant.

   - Dice the avocado and halve the cherry tomatoes.

2. **Assemble the Meditation Bowl:**
   - In a bowl, arrange the cooked quinoa, steamed broccoli, sliced carrots, diced avocado, and cherry tomatoes in a visually pleasing manner.

3. **Add Sesame Seeds:**
   - Sprinkle sesame seeds over the bowl for added texture and flavor.

4. **Garnish:**
   - Garnish with fresh cilantro to enhance the aroma and add a burst of freshness.

5. **Mindful Eating Ritual:**
   - Before diving in, take a moment to appreciate the colors, textures, and arrangement of the ingredients.

   - Inhale deeply and savor the aroma of the dish.

6. **Slow Bites:**
   - Take slow, deliberate bites, paying attention to the taste and texture of each component.

7. **Chew Mindfully:**
   - Chew each bite thoroughly, focusing on the sensations in your mouth.

8. **Pause Between Bites:**
   - Put down your utensils between bites and pause, allowing yourself to fully experience the flavors.

Benefits:

1. **Increased Satisfaction:** Mindful eating encourages a deeper appreciation of each bite, leading to increased satisfaction with your meal.

2. **Enhanced Digestion:** Chewing food thoroughly and savoring each bite aids digestion and nutrient absorption.

3. **Reduced Overeating:** Mindful eating helps prevent overeating by promoting awareness of hunger and fullness cues.

4. **Connection with Food:** Engaging your senses fosters a stronger connection with the food you eat, promoting a mindful relationship with nourishment.

5. **Stress Reduction:** The act of focusing on the present moment through mindful eating can contribute to stress reduction and improved overall well-being.

Application:

- **Daily Ritual:** Turn one meal each day into a mindful eating ritual, allowing yourself the time to truly savor and enjoy your food.

- **Social Gatherings:** Practice mindful eating during social gatherings, appreciating the shared experience of a meal with friends and family.

- **Portable Mindfulness:** Apply mindful eating practices to quick snacks or meals on-the-go, even if it's just a piece of fruit or a handful of nuts.

The Mindful Eating Meditation Bowl serves as a recipe for a mindful and intentional eating experience. It's a practice that can be applied to various meals, contributing to a healthier relationship with food and a more mindful approach to nourishment.

Quinoa and Kale Alkaline Power Bowl

Ingredients:
- 1 cup cooked quinoa
- 2 cups kale, chopped
- 1 cup cucumber, sliced
- 1 cup cherry tomatoes, halved
- 1/2 avocado, sliced
- 1/4 cup pumpkin seeds
- Lemon-tahini dressing (2 tablespoons tahini, juice of 1 lemon, 1 clove garlic, salt, and pepper to taste)

Preparation:
1. **Prepare Quinoa:**
   - Cook quinoa according to package instructions.

2. **Massage Kale:**
   - In a bowl, massage the chopped kale with a drizzle of olive oil for a few minutes until it becomes tender.

3. **Assemble the Power Bowl:**
   - In a large bowl, arrange the cooked quinoa, massaged kale, sliced

cucumber, halved cherry tomatoes, and sliced avocado.

4. **Top with Pumpkin Seeds:**
   - Sprinkle pumpkin seeds over the bowl for added crunch and nutritional benefits.

5. **Prepare Lemon-Tahini Dressing:**
   - In a small bowl, whisk together tahini, lemon juice, minced garlic, salt, and pepper to create a creamy dressing.

6. **Drizzle Dressing:**
   - Drizzle the lemon-tahini dressing over the power bowl.

7. **Toss Gently:**
   - Gently toss the ingredients to coat them evenly with the dressing.

Benefits:
1. **Alkaline Balance:** Kale, cucumber, and lemon are alkaline-forming foods, helping to maintain the body's pH balance.

2. **Nutrient-Rich:** This power bowl is packed with essential nutrients, including fiber, vitamins, minerals, and healthy fats from avocado and pumpkin seeds.

3. **Anti-Inflammatory:** Alkaline foods are often associated with an anti-inflammatory effect, which can help reduce inflammation in the body.

4. **Digestive Health:** Quinoa provides a good source of fiber, promoting digestive health and regular bowel movements.

5. **Satiety and Energy:** The combination of quinoa, kale, and healthy fats from avocado and pumpkin seeds provides lasting energy and a satisfying meal.

Application:
- **Lunch or Dinner Option:** Enjoy the Quinoa and Kale Alkaline Power Bowl as a wholesome lunch or dinner option.

- **Meal Prep:** This recipe is suitable for meal prepping, allowing you to have a nutritious and alkaline-balancing meal ready to go.

- **Customization:** Feel free to customize the ingredients based on personal preferences and seasonal availability of alkaline foods.

The Quinoa and Kale Alkaline Power Bowl serves as a recipe for a nourishing, alkaline-focused meal. It's a versatile and tasty way to incorporate alkaline foods into your diet, supporting overall health and vitality.

Calming Herbal Infusion

Ingredients:
- 1 tablespoon dried chamomile flowers
- 1 tablespoon dried lavender buds
- 1 teaspoon dried lemon balm leaves
- Honey or agave syrup (optional, for sweetness)
- Lemon slices (optional, for garnish)

Preparation:
1. **Boil Water:**
   - Bring 2 cups of water to a boil in a kettle or on the stovetop.

2. **Prepare Herbal Blend:**
   - In a teapot or heatproof pitcher, combine chamomile flowers, lavender buds, and lemon balm leaves.

3. **Pour Hot Water:**
   - Pour the boiling water over the herbal blend.

4. **Steep:**
   - Let the herbs steep for 5-7 minutes, allowing the flavors to infuse.

5. **Strain:**
   - If using loose herbs, strain the infusion to remove them.
6. **Sweeten and Garnish:**
   - Add honey or agave syrup for sweetness, if desired.

   - Garnish with lemon slices for a touch of freshness.

7. **Sip Mindfully:**
   - Find a quiet space, sip the herbal infusion slowly, and focus on the calming aroma and flavors.

Benefits:
1. **Caffeine-Free Relaxation:** This herbal infusion provides a caffeine-free alternative, ideal for winding down in the evening.

2. **Calming Herbs:** Chamomile, lavender, and lemon balm are known for their calming properties, promoting relaxation and reducing stress.

3. **Improved Sleep Quality:** Consuming caffeine-free herbal beverages in the evening may contribute to better sleep quality.

4. **Hydration:** Choosing herbal infusions supports hydration without the diuretic effects associated with caffeinated beverages.

5. **Mindful Ritual:** The act of preparing and enjoying a caffeine-free herbal infusion can become a mindful ritual, promoting a sense of calm and well-being.

Application:

- **Evening Ritual:** Incorporate this herbal infusion into your evening routine to signal the transition from a busy day to a restful evening.

- **Social Gatherings:** Share this calming ritual with friends or family during social gatherings for a serene and pleasant experience.

- **Post-Meal Beverage:** Enjoy this herbal infusion as a soothing post-meal beverage to aid digestion.

The Calming Herbal Infusion serves as a recipe for a caffeine-free and soothing beverage, providing a mindful alternative to traditional caffeinated drinks.

It's a simple and enjoyable way to limit caffeine intake, especially during the evening hours.

Homemade Greek Yogurt Parfait

Ingredients:
- 1 cup homemade or store-bought Greek yogurt
- 1/2 cup mixed berries (strawberries, blueberries, raspberries)
- 1 tablespoon honey or maple syrup
- 1/4 cup granola
- 1 tablespoon chia seeds
- A sprinkle of almonds or walnuts (optional)

Preparation:
1. **Prepare Greek Yogurt:**
   - If making yogurt at home, strain it to achieve a thicker Greek yogurt consistency.

2. **Layering the Parfait:**
   - In a glass or bowl, start with a layer of Greek yogurt.

3. **Add Berries:**
   - Add a layer of mixed berries on top of the yogurt.

4. **Drizzle Honey or Maple Syrup:**
   - Drizzle honey or maple syrup over the berries for natural sweetness.

5. **Sprinkle Granola:**
   - Sprinkle granola on top of the berries for crunch and additional fiber.

6. **Layer Chia Seeds:**
   - Add a layer of chia seeds for extra texture and a dose of omega-3 fatty acids.

7. **Repeat Layers:**
   - Repeat the layers until you reach the top of the glass or bowl.

8. **Finish with Nuts (Optional):**
   - If desired, top the parfait with a sprinkle of almonds or walnuts for added protein and healthy fats.

Benefits:
1. **Probiotic Boost:** Greek yogurt is rich in probiotics, beneficial bacteria that support a healthy gut microbiome.

2. **Antioxidant-Rich Berries:** Berries provide a powerful dose of antioxidants,

which contribute to overall health and well-being.

3. **Fiber from Granola:** The granola adds fiber to the parfait, supporting digestive health and promoting a feeling of fullness.

4. **Omega-3 Fatty Acids from Chia Seeds:** Chia seeds contribute omega-3 fatty acids, which have anti-inflammatory properties and support heart health.

5. **Natural Sweeteners:** Honey or maple syrup add sweetness without the refined sugars found in many commercial sweeteners.

Application:

- **Breakfast Option:** Enjoy this Greek Yogurt Parfait as a nutritious and satisfying breakfast option.

- **Snack Time:** It makes for a wholesome snack to curb midday cravings.

- **Dessert Alternative:** Serve the parfait as a healthier dessert option for a sweet ending to a meal.

The Homemade Greek Yogurt Parfait serves as a recipe for a delightful and probiotic-rich treat. It's a versatile dish that can be enjoyed at various times throughout the day, providing a tasty and nutritious way to support your gut health.

Creamy Almond Milk Chia Pudding

Ingredients:
- 1 cup unsweetened almond milk
- 1/4 cup chia seeds
- 1-2 tablespoons maple syrup or agave syrup
- 1/2 teaspoon vanilla extract
- Fresh berries for topping
- Chopped nuts for garnish (optional)

Preparation:
1. **Mix Almond Milk and Chia Seeds:**
   - In a bowl, combine almond milk, chia seeds, maple syrup (or agave syrup), and vanilla extract.

2. **Stir Well:**
   - Mix the ingredients thoroughly to ensure the chia seeds are well distributed.

3. **Refrigerate:**
   - Cover the bowl and refrigerate the mixture for at least 2 hours or overnight to allow the chia seeds to absorb the liquid and create a pudding-like consistency.

4. **Stir Again:**
   - Before serving, give the mixture a good stir to break up any clumps and achieve a smooth texture.

5. **Top with Berries and Nuts:**
   - Spoon the chia pudding into serving bowls or jars.
   - Top with fresh berries and, if desired, garnish with chopped nuts for added crunch.

Benefits:
1. **Dairy-Free:** Almond milk serves as a dairy alternative suitable for those who are lactose intolerant or follow a plant-based diet.

2. **Omega-3 Fatty Acids:** Chia seeds are rich in omega-3 fatty acids, supporting heart health and providing anti-inflammatory benefits.

3. **Low in Added Sugar:** Maple syrup or agave syrup adds sweetness without excessive refined sugars, making it a healthier alternative.

4. **Plant-Based Protein:** Chia seeds offer plant-based protein, contributing to a well-balanced and satisfying treat.

5. **Customizable:** This recipe is highly customizable – adjust sweetness, add spices like cinnamon, or experiment with different toppings to suit your preferences.

Application:

- **Breakfast Option:** Enjoy the Creamy Almond Milk Chia Pudding as a nutritious and filling breakfast option.

- **Snack Time:** It makes for a delightful and energy-boosting snack during the day.

- **Dessert Replacement:** Serve the chia pudding as a healthier alternative to traditional desserts after a meal.

The Creamy Almond Milk Chia Pudding is a testament to the versatility and deliciousness of dairy alternatives, offering a plant-based option that doesn't compromise on taste or texture.

It's a delightful treat that can be enjoyed at various times, providing a wholesome and satisfying experience.

Quinoa and Roasted Vegetable Buddha Bowl

Ingredients:
- 1 cup cooked quinoa
- 1 cup broccoli florets
- 1 cup cherry tomatoes, halved
- 1/2 cup carrots, sliced
- 1/2 cup bell peppers, sliced
- 2 tablespoons olive oil
- Salt and pepper to taste
- 1/4 cup hummus
- Fresh herbs for garnish (such as parsley or cilantro)

Preparation:
1. **Preheat Oven:**
   - Preheat the oven to 400°F (200°C).

2. **Prepare Vegetables:**
   - In a bowl, toss broccoli, cherry tomatoes, carrots, and bell peppers with olive oil, salt, and pepper.

3. **Roast Vegetables:**
   - Spread the seasoned vegetables on a baking sheet and roast in the preheated oven for 20-25 minutes

or until they are tender and slightly caramelized.

4. **Assemble Buddha Bowl:**
   - In a bowl, arrange a serving of cooked quinoa and top it with the roasted vegetables.

5. **Add Hummus:**
   - Spoon a dollop of hummus on the side or in the center of the bowl.

6. **Garnish:**
   - Garnish with fresh herbs for a burst of flavor and additional nutrients.

Benefits:
1. **Low-Glycemic Ingredients:** Quinoa and vegetables in this Buddha Bowl are low-glycemic, preventing rapid spikes in blood sugar levels.

2. **Stable Energy Release:** Low-glycemic foods promote a slower and more stable release of glucose into the bloodstream, sustaining energy levels.

3. **Fiber-Rich Quinoa:** Quinoa is a good source of fiber, supporting digestive health and contributing to a feeling of fullness.

4. **Vitamins and Minerals:** The variety of colorful vegetables provides essential vitamins, minerals, and antioxidants for overall health.

5. **Balanced Macronutrients:** The combination of quinoa, vegetables, and hummus provides a balanced mix of carbohydrates, proteins, and healthy fats.

Application:
- **Lunch or Dinner Option:** Enjoy this Buddha Bowl as a wholesome and satisfying lunch or dinner.

- **Meal Prep:** It's suitable for meal prepping, allowing you to have a nutritious and low-glycemic meal ready to go.

- **Customization:** Feel free to customize the vegetables and herbs based on personal preferences and seasonal availability.

The Quinoa and Roasted Vegetable Buddha Bowl is a recipe for a nutrient-dense, low-glycemic meal that supports stable blood sugar levels and overall health. It's a versatile dish that aligns with a balanced and mindful approach to nutrition.

Grilled Chicken and Quinoa Stuffed Peppers

Ingredients:
- 4 large bell peppers (assorted colors)
- 1 cup cooked quinoa
- 1 cup grilled chicken breast, diced
- 1/2 cup black beans, drained and rinsed
- 1/2 cup corn kernels (fresh or frozen)
- 1/2 cup diced tomatoes
- 1/4 cup red onion, finely chopped
- 1 teaspoon cumin
- 1 teaspoon chili powder
- Salt and pepper to taste
- 1 cup shredded cheese (cheddar or Mexican blend)
- Fresh cilantro for garnish

Preparation:
1. **Preheat the Grill or Oven:**
   - Preheat a grill or oven to 400°F (200°C).

2. **Prepare Bell Peppers:**
   - Cut the tops off the bell peppers, remove seeds and membranes, and lightly brush the outside with olive oil.

3. **Grill or Roast Peppers:**
   - Grill the peppers for 5-7 minutes on each side or roast them in the oven for 15-20 minutes until they are slightly charred and tender.

4. **Prepare Filling:**
   - In a bowl, combine cooked quinoa, diced grilled chicken, black beans, corn, diced tomatoes, red onion, cumin, chili powder, salt, and pepper.

5. **Stuff Peppers:**
   - Stuff each grilled or roasted pepper with the quinoa and chicken mixture.

6. **Top with Cheese:**
   - Sprinkle shredded cheese on top of each stuffed pepper.

7. **Finish Cooking:**
   - Return the stuffed peppers to the grill or oven for an additional 5-7 minutes or until the cheese is melted and bubbly.

8. **Garnish and Serve:**
   - Garnish with fresh cilantro and serve the stuffed peppers hot.

Benefits:
1. **Portion Control:** Stuffed peppers provide built-in portion control, as each pepper serves as an individual serving.

2. **Balanced Nutrients:** The combination of quinoa, grilled chicken, beans, and vegetables offers a well-balanced mix of proteins, carbohydrates, and fiber.

3. **Low-Calorie Option:** This dish is relatively low in calories while providing essential nutrients, making it suitable for those aiming for weight management.

4. **Satiety:** The fiber content from quinoa and vegetables promotes a feeling of fullness, supporting portion control.

5. **Versatility:** This recipe can be easily adapted to include other vegetables and lean proteins, catering to individual preferences.

Application:
- **Weeknight Dinner:** Enjoy the Grilled Chicken and Quinoa Stuffed Peppers as a

wholesome and portion-controlled weeknight dinner.

- **Meal Prep:** Make a batch of stuffed peppers for meal prepping, ensuring controlled portions for lunches or dinners throughout the week.

- **Social Gatherings:** Serve these stuffed peppers at gatherings as individual portions, allowing guests to enjoy a flavorful dish without overindulging.

This recipe exemplifies how flavorful and satisfying meals can be achieved while practicing portion control.

The Grilled Chicken and Quinoa Stuffed Peppers are not only delicious but also a practical way to manage portion sizes in a mindful and enjoyable manner.

Soothing Chamomile and Mint Herbal Tea Blend

Ingredients:
- 1 tablespoon dried chamomile flowers
- 1 tablespoon dried peppermint leaves
- Honey or lemon slices for optional sweetness and flavor

Preparation:
1. **Boil Water:**
   - Bring 2 cups of water to a boil in a kettle or on the stovetop.

2. **Prepare Herbal Blend:**
   - In a teapot or heatproof mug, combine dried chamomile flowers and dried peppermint leaves.

3. **Pour Hot Water:**
   - Pour the boiling water over the herbal blend.

4. **Steep:**
   - Let the herbs steep for 5-7 minutes, allowing the flavors to meld and infuse into the water.

5. **Strain:**
   - If using loose herbs, strain the tea to remove them.

6. **Sweeten and Flavor (Optional):**
   - Add honey or a few slices of lemon if you prefer a touch of sweetness or additional flavor.

7. **Enjoy Mindfully:**
   - Find a quiet space, sip the herbal tea slowly, and allow the calming aroma and warmth to envelop you.

Benefits:
1. **Calming Chamomile:** Chamomile is known for its calming and soothing properties, promoting relaxation and reducing stress.

2. **Refreshing Mint:** Peppermint adds a refreshing and invigorating element, aiding digestion and providing a burst of flavor.

3. **Digestive Support:** Both chamomile and mint are known for their digestive benefits, helping to alleviate indigestion and bloating.

4. **Caffeine-Free:** Herbal teas are naturally caffeine-free, making them suitable for evening consumption without disrupting sleep.
5. **Hydration:** Sipping on herbal tea contributes to overall hydration, supporting various bodily functions.

Application:
- **Evening Ritual:** Incorporate this herbal tea into your evening routine to unwind and signal the transition to a restful night.

- **Stressful Days:** Enjoy a cup of this soothing blend during stressful moments or busy days to promote relaxation.

- **Social Sharing:** Share this herbal tea with friends or family during social gatherings for a calming and enjoyable experience.

The Soothing Chamomile and Mint Herbal Tea Blend serves as a simple yet effective recipe for creating a tranquil and enjoyable tea-drinking experience.

It's a versatile beverage that can be enjoyed in various settings, providing a moment of calm and well-being.

Citrus Infused Spa Water

Ingredients:
- 1 lemon, sliced
- 1 lime, sliced
- 1 orange, sliced
- Fresh mint leaves
- 2 liters of filtered water
- Ice cubes (optional)

Preparation:
1. **Prepare Citrus Slices:**
   - Wash and slice the lemon, lime, and orange into thin rounds.

2. **Assemble Ingredients:**
   - In a large pitcher, combine the citrus slices and a handful of fresh mint leaves.

3. **Add Water:**
   - Pour 2 liters of filtered water into the pitcher.

4. **Refrigerate:**
   - Place the pitcher in the refrigerator and let it chill for at least 2 hours or overnight to allow the flavors to infuse.

5. **Serve Over Ice (Optional):**
   - When ready to serve, you can add ice cubes to individual glasses for an extra refreshing touch.

6. **Garnish (Optional):**
   - Garnish each glass with a sprig of fresh mint for a visually appealing presentation.

7. **Stay Hydrated:**
   - Sip on this citrus-infused spa water throughout the day to stay hydrated and refreshed.

Benefits:
1. **Hydration Support:** The main ingredient is water, providing essential hydration to support bodily functions and overall well-being.

2. **Natural Electrolytes:** Citrus fruits contain electrolytes like potassium, which aids in hydration and helps maintain a healthy balance of fluids in the body.

3. **Antioxidant Boost:** Citrus fruits are rich in antioxidants, which help combat free radicals and contribute to skin health.

4. **Minty Freshness:** Fresh mint not only adds a burst of flavor but also has

digestive benefits and may contribute to a sense of alertness.

5. **Zero Calories:** This infused water is calorie-free, making it a healthy alternative to sugary beverages.

Application:

- **Daily Hydration:** Make Citrus Infused Spa Water your go-to daily hydration choice for a flavorful and enjoyable drink.

- **Outdoor Activities:** Bring a chilled pitcher to outdoor gatherings, picnics, or workouts to stay cool and hydrated.

- **Hydration Reminder:** Keep a pitcher in the fridge as a visual reminder to prioritize hydration throughout the day.

The Citrus Infused Spa Water is a simple and effective recipe to elevate your hydration routine. It's a versatile and enjoyable beverage suitable for various occasions, making the act of staying hydrated a delightful and refreshing experience.

Balanced Buddha Bowl for Intermittent Fasting

Ingredients:

- 1 cup cooked quinoa
- 4 ounces grilled chicken breast or tofu
- 1 cup steamed broccoli
- 1/2 avocado, sliced
- 1/4 cup shredded carrots
- 2 tablespoons hummus
- Lemon-tahini dressing (2 tablespoons tahini, juice of 1 lemon, salt, and pepper to taste)
- Fresh herbs for garnish (such as cilantro or parsley)

Preparation:

1. **Cook Quinoa:**
   - Prepare 1 cup of quinoa according to package instructions.

2. **Grill Chicken or Tofu:**
   - Grill 4 ounces of chicken breast or tofu until fully cooked.

3. **Steam Broccoli:**
   - Steam 1 cup of broccoli until tender but still vibrant.

4. **Assemble Buddha Bowl:**
   * In a bowl, arrange cooked quinoa, grilled chicken or tofu, steamed broccoli, sliced avocado, shredded carrots, and hummus.

5. **Prepare Lemon-Tahini Dressing:**
   * In a small bowl, whisk together tahini, lemon juice, salt, and pepper.

6. **Drizzle Dressing:**
   * Drizzle the lemon-tahini dressing over the Buddha bowl.

7. **Garnish:**
   * Garnish with fresh herbs for added flavor.

Benefits:

1. **Nutrient-Rich Ingredients:** The Buddha bowl includes a mix of whole grains, lean protein, and a variety of colorful vegetables, providing a range of essential nutrients.

2. **Satiety and Fullness:** The combination of protein, fiber, and healthy fats promotes a feeling of fullness and satisfaction during the fasting window.

3. **Stable Blood Sugar Levels:** The balanced macronutrient profile helps stabilize blood sugar levels, supporting energy levels and mental clarity during fasting periods.

4. **Customizable:** The recipe is easily customizable based on individual preferences and dietary restrictions.

5. **Hydration:** The hydrating vegetables and lemon-tahini dressing contribute to overall hydration.

Application:
- **Breaking the Fast:** Enjoy this Balanced Buddha Bowl as a nutrient-dense meal to break your fast during the eating window.

- **Lunch or Dinner:** Incorporate this recipe into your lunch or dinner rotation to maintain balanced and healthy eating habits.

- **Meal Prep:** Prepare components of the Buddha bowl in advance for easy meal prepping during the fasting period.

This Balanced Buddha Bowl is designed to align with the principles of intermittent fasting, providing a well-rounded and satisfying meal to support overall health and wellness. It's a versatile recipe that can be adapted to various dietary preferences and fasting schedules.

Fresh and Vibrant Mediterranean Salad

Ingredients:
- 2 cups mixed greens (spinach, kale, arugula)
- 1 cup cherry tomatoes, halved
- 1 cucumber, sliced
- 1/2 red onion, thinly sliced
- 1/2 cup Kalamata olives, pitted
- 1/2 cup feta cheese, crumbled
- 1/4 cup extra-virgin olive oil
- 2 tablespoons balsamic vinegar
- 1 teaspoon Dijon mustard
- 1 clove garlic, minced
- Salt and pepper to taste
- Fresh basil leaves for garnish

Preparation:
1. **Prepare the Dressing:**
   - In a small bowl, whisk together extra-virgin olive oil, balsamic vinegar, Dijon mustard, minced garlic, salt, and pepper. Set aside.

2. **Assemble the Salad:**
   - In a large bowl, combine mixed greens, cherry tomatoes,

cucumber, red onion, Kalamata olives, and crumbled feta cheese.

3. **Drizzle with Dressing:**
   - Drizzle the prepared dressing over the salad and toss gently to coat the ingredients evenly.

4. **Garnish:**
   - Garnish the salad with fresh basil leaves for a burst of flavor and aroma.

Benefits:

1. **Nutrient-Rich Ingredients:** The salad incorporates a variety of colorful vegetables, providing essential vitamins, minerals, and antioxidants.

2. **Healthy Fats:** Extra-virgin olive oil and feta cheese contribute healthy fats, supporting heart health and overall well-being.

3. **Low Processed Content:** By focusing on whole, unprocessed ingredients, this salad minimizes reliance on processed foods, which often contain added sugars, preservatives, and unhealthy fats.

4. **Dietary Fiber:** The combination of greens, vegetables, and olives provides

dietary fiber, promoting digestive health and a feeling of fullness.

5. **Versatile and Customizable:** The recipe is versatile, allowing for customization based on personal preferences and seasonal availability of ingredients.

Application:

- **Lunch or Dinner Option:** Enjoy the Fresh and Vibrant Mediterranean Salad as a satisfying and wholesome lunch or dinner.

- **Social Gatherings:** Share this nutrient-packed salad at social gatherings, promoting a healthy and delicious option for friends and family.

- **Meal Prep:** Prepare components of the salad in advance for convenient meal prepping during busy days.

This Mediterranean Salad serves as a recipe for a nutrient-dense and unprocessed meal, aligning with the goal of limiting processed foods and embracing a whole-foods approach to nutrition. It's a flavorful and satisfying dish that supports overall health and well-being.

Avocado and Salmon Quinoa Bowl

Ingredients:
- 1 cup cooked quinoa
- 4 ounces grilled or baked salmon fillet, flaked
- 1 ripe avocado, sliced
- 1 cup cherry tomatoes, halved
- 1/4 cup red onion, finely chopped
- 2 tablespoons extra-virgin olive oil
- 1 tablespoon balsamic vinegar
- 1 teaspoon Dijon mustard
- Salt and pepper to taste
- Fresh dill for garnish

Preparation:
1. **Prepare Quinoa:**
   - Cook 1 cup of quinoa according to package instructions.

2. **Cook Salmon:**
   - Grill or bake the salmon fillet until fully cooked. Flake the salmon into bite-sized pieces.

3. **Assemble Quinoa Bowl:**
   - In a bowl, arrange the cooked quinoa, flaked salmon, sliced avocado, cherry tomatoes, and chopped red onion.

4. **Prepare Dressing:**
   - In a small bowl, whisk together extra-virgin olive oil, balsamic vinegar, Dijon mustard, salt, and pepper.

5. **Drizzle Dressing:**
   - Drizzle the dressing over the quinoa bowl.

6. **Garnish:**
   - Garnish with fresh dill for a touch of herbaceous flavor.

Benefits:
1. **Omega-3 Fatty Acids:** Salmon is rich in omega-3 fatty acids, supporting heart health, brain function, and reducing inflammation.

2. **Monounsaturated Fats:** Avocado provides monounsaturated fats, which contribute to heart health and may help lower bad cholesterol levels.

3. **Healthy Cooking Oil:** Extra-virgin olive oil is a source of monounsaturated fats and polyphenols, providing anti-inflammatory benefits.
4. **Protein and Fiber:** Quinoa offers a combination of protein and fiber, promoting satiety and digestive health.
5. **Antioxidant-Rich Vegetables:** Cherry tomatoes and red onion provide antioxidants, supporting overall health and protecting cells from damage.

Application:

- **Lunch or Dinner Option:** Enjoy the Avocado and Salmon Quinoa Bowl as a nourishing and satiating meal for lunch or dinner.

- **Post-Workout Meal:** Incorporate this recipe into your post-workout routine to replenish protein and healthy fats.

- **Meal Prep:** Prepare components of the quinoa bowl in advance for convenient and healthy meal prepping.

This Avocado and Salmon Quinoa Bowl is a celebration of healthy fats, offering a delicious and satisfying way to incorporate omega-3 fatty acids and monounsaturated fats into your diet.

Colorful Chickpea and Vegetable Stir-Fry

Ingredients:

- 1 can (15 ounces) chickpeas, drained and rinsed
- 2 cups broccoli florets
- 1 bell pepper (any color), thinly sliced
- 1 carrot, julienned
- 1 cup snap peas, ends trimmed
- 3 cloves garlic, minced
- 2 tablespoons olive oil
- 2 tablespoons soy sauce (or tamari for a gluten-free option)
- 1 tablespoon honey or maple syrup
- 1 teaspoon grated ginger
- 1 tablespoon sesame seeds (optional)
- Brown rice or quinoa for serving

Preparation:

1. **Stir-Fry Vegetables:**
   - Heat olive oil in a large pan or wok over medium-high heat. Add broccoli, bell pepper, carrot, and snap peas. Stir-fry for 5-7 minutes until the vegetables are tender-crisp.

2. **Add Chickpeas:**
   - Add the drained chickpeas to the pan and cook for an additional 2-3 minutes to heat through.

3. **Prepare Sauce:**
   - In a small bowl, whisk together soy sauce, honey (or maple syrup), and grated ginger.

4. **Combine and Toss:**
   - Pour the sauce over the vegetables and chickpeas. Add minced garlic and toss everything together until well-coated and heated through.

5. **Serve:**
   - Serve the colorful stir-fry over brown rice or quinoa.

6. **Garnish (Optional):**
   - Sprinkle sesame seeds on top for added crunch and flavor.

Benefits:

1. **Rich in Dietary Fiber:** Chickpeas and vegetables are excellent sources of dietary fiber, promoting digestive regularity and a healthy gut.

2. **Nutrient Variety:** The colorful array of vegetables provides a diverse range of vitamins, minerals, and antioxidants.
3. **Protein Boost:** Chickpeas contribute plant-based protein, making this stir-fry a satisfying and balanced meal.

4. **Low in Saturated Fat:** This recipe is low in saturated fat, supporting heart health.

5. **Customizable:** Easily customize the stir-fry with additional veggies or your favorite protein source.

Application:
- **Weeknight Dinner:** Enjoy the Colorful Chickpea and Vegetable Stir-Fry as a quick and nutritious weeknight dinner.

- **Meal Prep:** Prepare a batch for meal prepping, ensuring a convenient and healthy option for lunches.

- **Plant-Based Option:** This fiber-rich dish is suitable for those seeking a plant-based or vegetarian meal.

The Colorful Chickpea and Vegetable Stir-Fry celebrates the abundance of fiber-rich foods, offering a flavorful and satisfying way to prioritize digestive health while enjoying a delicious meal.

Rainbow Veggie Quinoa Bowl

Ingredients:
- 1 cup quinoa, rinsed
- 2 cups water or vegetable broth (for cooking quinoa)
- 1 tablespoon olive oil
- 1 red bell pepper, thinly sliced
- 1 yellow bell pepper, thinly sliced
- 1 orange bell pepper, thinly sliced
- 1 zucchini, sliced into half-moons
- 1 cup cherry tomatoes, halved
- 1 cup purple cabbage, thinly shredded
- 1 cup baby spinach leaves
- 1/4 cup fresh cilantro, chopped
- 1/4 cup feta cheese, crumbled (optional)
- Balsamic vinaigrette or lemon-tahini dressing for drizzling

Preparation:
1. **Cook Quinoa:**
   - In a saucepan, combine quinoa and water or vegetable broth. Bring to a boil, then reduce heat, cover, and simmer for 15-20 minutes or until quinoa is cooked and water is absorbed. Fluff with a fork.

2. **Sauté Vegetables:**
   - In a large skillet, heat olive oil over medium heat. Add red, yellow, and orange bell peppers, zucchini, and cherry tomatoes. Sauté for 5-7 minutes until vegetables are tender-crisp.

3. **Assemble the Bowl:**
   - In serving bowls, layer cooked quinoa with sautéed vegetables, purple cabbage, baby spinach, and fresh cilantro.

4. **Optional Toppings:**
   - Sprinkle crumbled feta cheese on top for added creaminess.

5. **Drizzle Dressing:**
   - Drizzle balsamic vinaigrette or lemon-tahini dressing over the bowl for extra flavor.

Benefits:
1. **Diverse Nutrients:** Each colorful vegetable contributes a unique set of vitamins, minerals, and antioxidants, promoting overall health.

2. **Dietary Fiber:** The combination of quinoa and a variety of vegetables provides dietary fiber, supporting digestive health.
3. **Low-Calorie Option:** This veggie-packed bowl is low in calories while being rich in volume, making it a suitable option for those aiming for weight management.

4. **Plant-Based Goodness:** The recipe is naturally plant-based, catering to individuals with vegetarian or vegan dietary preferences.

5. **Customizable:** Adapt the bowl based on seasonal availability and personal taste preferences.

Application:
- **Lunch or Dinner:** Enjoy the Rainbow Veggie Quinoa Bowl as a vibrant and nutritious lunch or dinner option.

- **Meal Prep:** Prepare components of the bowl in advance for convenient and healthy meal prepping during busy days.

- **Social Sharing:** Share this colorful and nutrient-packed dish at gatherings, promoting a wholesome and visually appealing dining experience.

Lemon-Dill Baked Salmon with Quinoa and Roasted Vegetables

Ingredients:
* 4 salmon fillets (6 ounces each)
* 1 cup quinoa, rinsed
* 2 cups water or vegetable broth (for cooking quinoa)
* 1 bunch asparagus, trimmed
* 1 cup cherry tomatoes, halved
* 1 tablespoon olive oil
* Salt and pepper to taste
* Zest of 1 lemon
* 2 tablespoons fresh dill, chopped
* Lemon wedges for serving

Preparation:
1. **Preheat Oven:**
   * Preheat the oven to 400°F (200°C).

2. **Bake Salmon:**
   * Place salmon fillets on a baking sheet lined with parchment paper. Season with salt, pepper, and lemon zest. Bake for 15-20 minutes or until the salmon flakes easily with a fork.

3. **Roast Vegetables:**
   - On a separate baking sheet, toss asparagus and cherry tomatoes with olive oil, salt, and pepper. Roast in the oven for 15-20 minutes or until vegetables are tender.

4. **Cook Quinoa:**
   - In a saucepan, combine quinoa and water or vegetable broth. Bring to a boil, then reduce heat, cover, and simmer for 15-20 minutes or until quinoa is cooked. Fluff with a fork.

5. **Assemble the Plate:**
   - Arrange a serving of quinoa on each plate. Top with baked salmon fillet and roasted vegetables.

6. **Sprinkle with Fresh Dill:**
   - Sprinkle fresh dill over the salmon and vegetables for added flavor.

7. **Serve with Lemon Wedges:**
   - Serve the dish with lemon wedges on the side for a citrusy touch.

Benefits:
1. **Omega-3 Fatty Acids:** Salmon is rich in omega-3 fatty acids, promoting heart health and reducing inflammation.

2. **Complete Protein Source:** Salmon provides high-quality protein, essential for muscle repair and overall body function.

3. **Quinoa's Nutrient Profile:** Quinoa is a nutrient-dense grain, offering a complete protein source, fiber, and various vitamins and minerals.

4. **Antioxidant-Rich Vegetables:** Asparagus and cherry tomatoes contribute antioxidants, supporting overall health.

5. **Herbaceous Flavor:** Fresh dill adds a burst of herbaceous flavor while offering additional antioxidants.

Application:

- **Dinner Delight:** Enjoy this Lemon-Dill Baked Salmon with Quinoa and Roasted Vegetables as a flavorful and nutritious dinner option.

- **Special Occasions:** Serve this dish at special occasions or gatherings to impress guests with a delicious and health-conscious meal.

- **Weekly Rotation:** Make it a regular part of your weekly meal rotation to consistently incorporate omega-3 rich foods into your diet.

Grilled Chicken and Quinoa Salad with Avocado-Lime Dressing

Ingredients:

For the Salad:
- 1 cup quinoa, rinsed
- 2 cups water or chicken broth (for cooking quinoa)
- 4 boneless, skinless chicken breasts
- 1 tablespoon olive oil
- Salt and pepper to taste
- 6 cups mixed salad greens
- 1 cucumber, sliced
- 1 cup cherry tomatoes, halved
- 1/4 cup red onion, thinly sliced
- 1/4 cup feta cheese, crumbled (optional)
- 1/4 cup almonds, sliced and toasted

For the Avocado-Lime Dressing:
- 1 ripe avocado
- Juice of 2 limes
- 2 tablespoons olive oil
- 1 clove garlic, minced
- Salt and pepper to taste
- 2 tablespoons fresh cilantro, chopped

Preparation:

1. Cook Quinoa:

- In a saucepan, combine quinoa and water or chicken broth. Bring to a boil, then reduce heat, cover, and simmer for 15-20 minutes or until quinoa is cooked. Fluff with a fork.

2. Grill Chicken:

- Preheat the grill. Brush chicken breasts with olive oil and season with salt and pepper. Grill for 6-8 minutes per side or until cooked through. Let it rest for a few minutes before slicing.

3. Prepare Avocado-Lime Dressing:

- In a blender or food processor, combine avocado, lime juice, olive oil, minced garlic, salt, pepper, and chopped cilantro. Blend until smooth.

4. Assemble the Salad:

- In a large bowl, combine cooked quinoa, sliced grilled chicken, mixed salad greens, cucumber, cherry tomatoes, and red onion.

5. **Drizzle with Dressing:**
   - Drizzle the avocado-lime dressing over the salad and toss gently to coat.

6. **Top with Toppings:**
   - Sprinkle crumbled feta cheese (optional) and toasted sliced almonds on top for added flavor and texture.

Benefits:
1. **High-Quality Protein:** Grilled chicken provides a lean and high-quality protein source, essential for muscle health and repair.

2. **Quinoa's Nutrient Profile:** Quinoa offers a complete protein source along with fiber, vitamins, and minerals.

3. **Healthy Fats:** The avocado-lime dressing contributes heart-healthy fats, enhancing flavor and nutritional value.

4. **Nutrient-Rich Vegetables:** Mixed greens, cucumber, cherry tomatoes, and red onion provide a variety of vitamins, minerals, and antioxidants.

5. **Satisfying and Flavorful:** The combination of textures and flavors, including feta cheese and toasted almonds, makes this salad satisfying and delicious.

Application:

- **Lunch or Dinner:** Enjoy this Grilled Chicken and Quinoa Salad as a wholesome and satisfying lunch or dinner option.

- **Post-Workout Meal:** Incorporate this protein-packed dish into your post-workout routine to support muscle recovery.

- **Meal Prep:** Prepare components in advance for easy meal prepping during busy weekdays.

This Grilled Chicken and Quinoa Salad with Avocado-Lime Dressing exemplifies how a lean protein focus can be both nutritious and delightful.

It's a versatile recipe suitable for various occasions and contributes to a balanced and protein-rich diet.

CONCLUSION

As you get to the end of The Ultimate Galveston Diet, you'll have discovered the power of feeding your body, balancing hormones, and adopting a lifestyle that goes beyond typical dieting.

You've not only lost healthy weight but also gained a thorough grasp of the complex relationship between your body and hormones as a result of this comprehensive program.

As you reflect on your accomplishments, keep in mind that The Ultimate Galveston Diet is more than simply a quick fix; it's a plan for a healthy, balanced life. The habits you've developed, the healthy meals you've consumed, and the mindful practices you've adopted are the foundation for a healthier, more vibrant self.

Your success is evaluated not only by the number on the scale, but also by the renewed energy, confidence, and vitality that emanates from inside.

The spirit of rebirth in Galveston has become a part of your journey, reminding you that every day is an opportunity to prioritize your well-being and enjoy life to the fullest.

The Ultimate Galveston Diet isn't simply a phase in your life; it's a way of life that you may live for years to come. Continue to enjoy nutrient-rich meals, engage in revitalizing activities, and cultivate self-care routines that benefit your overall health.

Carry with you the lessons acquired from this trip, as well as the resilience that comes with prioritizing your health, as you go ahead.

Celebrate your accomplishments, remember the lessons you've learned, and know that The Ultimate Galveston Diet has given you the skills you need to travel your health path with confidence and purpose.

Your dedication to a balanced life and harmonious hormonal health demonstrates your commitment to a better and healthier self.

May the vitality of Galveston linger with you, motivating you to make conscious decisions, prioritize self-care, and thrive on your journey to long-term well-being.

This isn't the end; it's the start of a new chapter, one filled with vitality, harmony, and the bright energy that comes from living your healthiest, happiest life.

Congrats on finishing The Ultimate Galveston Diet!

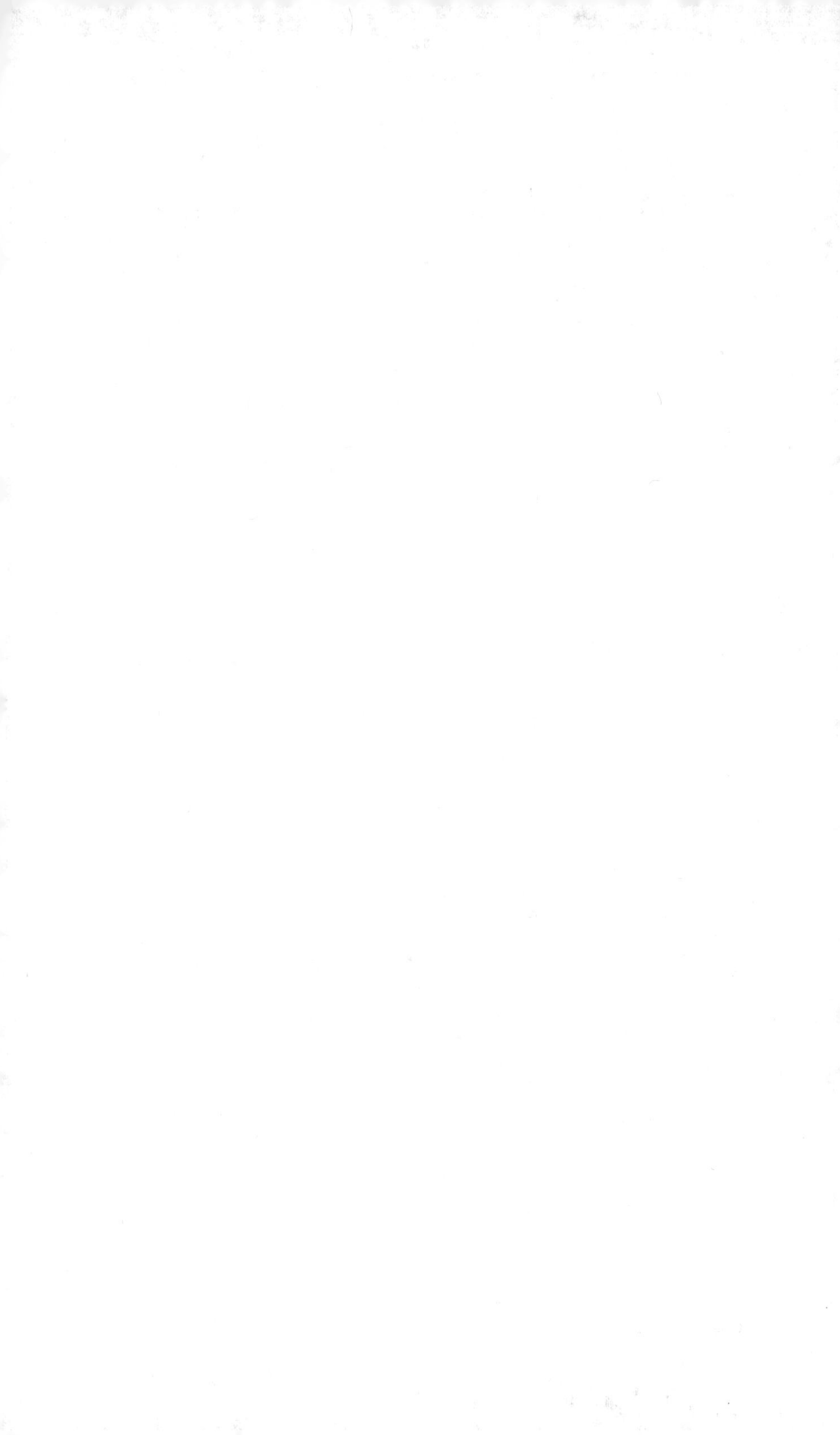